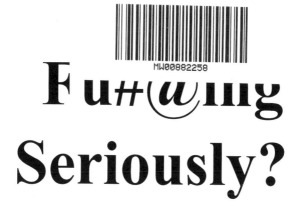

Fu#@ing Seriously?

Real NSFW Stories from a Small-Town ER

Kerry Hamm

Disclaimer:

Names, locations, and portions of the details included in this book have been altered to protect the privacy of those involved.

Edited for quality purposes after release.

NOTICE: I cannot stress this introduction enough, whether you have or have not read my other books. This entire book is a special not-safe-for-work edition filled with filthy language, overly-sarcastic (and sometimes mean-spirited) observations and commentary regarding patients and the hospital itself. This material may not be suitable for all audiences, so if you are offended by the excessive use of curse words, judgmental criticisms, or dark humor, feel free to stop here.

Now, if you wish to continue with stories that WILL appear in another safe-for-work version of this series released at the same time, I'll continue with my usual lead-in, which is similar to the following:

If you haven't read the first six books, don't worry. Let me fill you in on a few things, including those that have changed since the last edition:

Welcome to a small-town Emergency Room in Ohio. With six trauma bays, one mental health room, one low pressure room, one quarantine room, and 11 other exam bays, this ER has the capacity to fit 21 patients at a time, with more than 100 patients often lining up in the lobby and waiting room on any given evening shift.

We're no big-shot inner city hospital. We transfer out burns and severe pediatric cases. We have a mental health floor, inpatient rehab, intermediate care/critical care, and hospice floor in addition to pediatrics, general surgery, obstetrics, and nursery floors. Unless patients are directly admitted from facilities in surrounding areas, they show up in our department first.

My name is Kerry and I'm the first person you'll see when you come through those ER doors: registration.

On any given day, two to three clerks work during the day and evening shifts, taking turns gathering names, birth dates, and chief complaints at the front (while juggling floor transfers, admits from surrounding hospitals, and outside phone calls from some cat lady named Linda who's making her third call this shift to see if we think she needs to come in for tingling in her left butt cheek), and then in the back, where we enter patients' rooms to gather contact and insurance information to complete the registration process.

It used to be, once 11 p.m. hit, I waved to my coworkers as they walked out the door, and I was left at the registration desk with a triage nurse in a small room behind the desk, security lurking behind a two-way mirror that takes up an entire wall in front of the registration desk, a not-so-empty waiting room to my right, and six registered nurses and one or two doctors in the back.

Someone was listening and gave me a coworker to help get through the nights, but that bum up and quit to go to a less stressful department. (This person knows I mean this in a joking manner; I want to clarify that to readers.) I miss my ex-coworker dearly, and my shifts just haven't been the same without our well-oiled teamwork.

When I first started the first book, I didn't think there would be a second. And then, the third was going to be 'the very last.' But then all hell broke loose one night, and I realized there's never going to be a shortage of stories.

Before I started writing these books, I didn't realize just how many crazy things I see on a daily basis. At times, I can clock out from a shift with three to five new stories to tell. I realized for being such a small hospital in a rural area, this place sees quite a few off-the-wall events/people. My friends encouraged me to tell the stories, and here we are.

Every story here is true, though dialogue has been changed slightly, all names have been changed, and some situations have been slightly altered to protect patient privacy. It has never been my intention to exploit the heartaches or embarrassments of others, but simply offer a glimpse into the world of the

Emergency Room, where every patient seems to be a wild card.

<u>Cheat Sheet</u>

Readers have brought to my attention that some of the terms I use in my books are confusing, meaning my readers can't fully enjoy the stories. I plan to edit my previous editions to include this 'cheat sheet' of terms I frequently use.

MVA: Motor Vehicle Accident

ETOH: ethyl alcohol is the real meaning of this, but in our ER this means our patient is drunk

CC/cc: chief complaint

Tones dropping: a series of melodic beeps play before dispatch alerts medics of a patient's call. Most of us groan when we hear the tones because we know we're getting another patient.

Stemi: a procedure in which a patient is taken to the Cath Lab to clear a cardiac blockage. From what I understand, this is done by making an incision near the groin rather than entering through the heart itself.

Face sheet/facesheet: a piece of paper detailing the patient's name, contact information, next of kin, primary physician, chief complaint, and insurance information. One copy must go to the back, the other to our tray. Then, another must go to medics, the floor (if a patient is admitted), and the coroner (if it comes down to that).

NOK: next of kin

DID: died in department

DOA: dead on arrival

BAC: blood alcohol content

Bus: another term for ambulance

If I have forgotten to include any terms you feel others may not recognize, feel free to leave a review with your suggestion!

While an RN was listening to a patient's heart and lungs, the **two-year-old** punched her in the nose with a closed fist and ordered, "Get away from me, bitch."

Welcome to the ER, folks—where patients and family members have no qualms about how you're verbally or physically abused on a daily basis, yet God forbid you ask them to wait three damn minutes!

<u>Play a Love Game</u>

The patient in this story appears in one of my previous books, and I highly doubt she *won't* appear again. She's one of those patients we recognize instantly and have to notify security about when she arrives because I think it must be impossible for her to go anyplace without bringing the bullshit with her.

To give a little backstory here, the patient was dating Man 1. Then she broke up with Man 1 so she could go back to Man 2, her ex-boyfriend. Well, she cheated on Man 2 with Man 3. When Man 2 found out the patient was banging every guy in town, he dumped her (again) and she found Man 4. She moved in with Man 4 within a week of meeting him and then went behind his back to screw Man 1. Incidentally, the woman's relationship status on Facebook for the longest time was, 'It's complicated.'

A few weeks later, the patient became engaged; not to Man 4, but to Man 1.

However, she was still living with Man 4, so this didn't blow over so well.

She came to the ER with Man 4 at her side and stated to me that she was in a physical altercation with her ex.

I swear, it took every muscle and thought in my mind not to ask, "Which one?" as she stood in front of me. But I didn't ask that because I'm a *professional*, damn it.

Our frequent flyer went to triage and then was taken to a non-trauma room. Man 4 accompanied the woman.

Not too much longer later, I went to the back and passed Man 4 as he was heading out to smoke. I then stopped at the nurses' station and handed off a few papers, but was stopped as I tried to go back to my desk.

"That man is not to come back here again," one of the doctors ordered me.

I nodded. "Okay."

"I mean it, Registration," he said sternly.

"Kerry."

"What?"

"Kerry. My name is Kerry."

He rolled his eyes and I was reminded of why all the staff back in the ER thought he was an asshole.

"Whatever," he said. "Just do your job and don't let him back."

I started to walk away when the charge nurse jogged up beside me.

"Hey, what did that patient in nine tell you when she registered?"

I shrugged. "Just that she got in a fight with her ex."

"Well," said the charge, "she just told us the guy with her beat the crap out of her and threatened to kill her if she told anyone. She's pressing charges, so the cops are on the way."

"Wow."

"Yeah," agreed the nurse. "Just tell him he can't come back and you don't know why."

I nodded.

Man 4 was waiting to get back to the ER when I reached my desk.

"Ready to go to her room again," he told me, as if nothing was the matter.

I shook my head and sat down. "They told me no visitors for a while."

"No visitors? But I came in with her. Why can't I go back?"

"Dunno," I said.

"Well if that's not a bunch of fucking bullshit," he said loudly, as he hit the desktop with the palm of his hand.

Then the man shook his head, too, and said calmly, "Okay then," before walking out the door.

I figured *he* figured out that the patient had ratted him out and wanted to get the hell out of Dodge before the cops showed up, so I went about minding my business.

The first cop to show up was my favorite: the woman all the angry drunks and druggies refer to as the 'bitch dyke' because of her pixie haircut and boxy figure. She's been mentioned in previous books, but if you've forgotten or haven't read those books, I'll give you a quick refresher. You don't fuck with this woman, like, at all. She's strong. She's fast. If you piss her off by running, she'll tackle your ass to the ground, and she'll clothesline you like you wanted to do to that one annoying kid when you played Red Rover. Seriously, she's the toughest cop I know, and she doesn't take shit from anyone.

"What are you doing here in the middle of the night? Didn't you go to days?" I casually asked.

She nodded. "Yeah, but I'm pulling a double. Tell me about what's going on."

I couldn't tell her much, so I directed her to the charge nurse.

Well, as she was in the back, another cop came in. This guy was from the county over, and I was confused as to why we now had two officers from two counties in our ER for one patient.

"She didn't know where the assault took place," explained the male officer, "because they were driving around."

Oh, okay. I guess that made a bit more sense.

Before I could open the door for him, the first cop came out to the lobby and tried to fill in the second.

But all her information was wrong.

"She just got engaged," the cop said, "and I guess he beat the crap out of her."

"Weird thing to do when you just get engaged," the second cop replied.

I interrupted and explained to both officers the love...rectangle?...going on in the patient's love life, and this somehow lead to the female officer ordering me with wide eyes to bring up the patient's Facebook page. And, well, who am I to deny a direct order from a cop?

She made the strangest expressions as I scrolled briskly down the patient's and boyfriends' walls, showing her nothing but a bunch of dramatic people tagging each other or memes like Kermit the Frog talking about eating someone out—sickening things, really, that I guess you could post on your Facebook wall, but it'd probably not be best to post them for the public to see in case, well, the cops want to look you up online or something. And I'm not supposed to admit this at all because it's a huge no-no in this industry, but people...if you come in and are a dick, we look you up on Facebook or type your name in Google, okay? Nurses do it. Doctors do it.

The cops obviously do it. We've even read live updates of how much a patient said she hated her 'lesbian' nurse in between the rounds the nurse made to the patient's room to make sure the woman got the 10,000 popsicles and sodas she asked for during the visit for menstrual cramps.

Anyway, once I explained the clusterfuck to the cops, they wanted to wait at the desk for an officer coming from Kentucky because the patient wasn't sure if the assault happened over state lines, but she was leaning towards yes more so than it occurring in the counties from which the other officers arrived.

Seriously.

Well, when the third officer arrived, the other two explained the situation and then went into detail about the patient's injuries. According to officers, the patient said Man 4 strangled her and she had the red marks on her neck as evidence of the abuse. Man 4 also struggled with the patient as he attempted to—and succeeded in—ripping the engagement ring from the patient's finger. He then hit her in places where someone could not see the bruises unless the patient was undressed or the skin was exposed, like her abdomen, her upper arms, and her back. The altercation allegedly began in the cab of the truck, but it eventually moved to the center of a country road.

Domestic violence against any gender is disgusting and is not the least bit funny, so I will make no jokes about this matter. I encourage anyone in an abusive relationship to seek help any way possible, and if you are approached by a victim of domestic violence, I hope you are able to provide assistance or direct the victim to someone who can.

To get on with the craziness of this situation, all three cops went back to the patient's room to confirm the story and injuries, as well as pin down a location by asking the patient about physical markers she may have noticed along the way.

Once this was all figured out, the officers returned to the desk and spoke about apprehending Man 4.

You know, it didn't take long for this to happen.

All three cops went to the parking lot, but I guess one of them noticed the man's truck was in our parking lot.

'Bitch dyke' came inside, laughing, and said, "I can't believe he's this fucking stupid."

I wasn't all that sure what she meant by that until she came back from the patient's room and explained to me that he made his girlfriend hold the keys to the truck and hadn't been able to retrieve them because we banned him from the back.

Thinking he had the perfect plan, this dumbass locked the doors to the truck, sprawled out flat on his back in the cab, and tried to hide from the cops.

But there was one thing that gave this man away.

See, he was smoking a cigarette and the driver's side window was cracked, so officers knew he was inside by the ribbons of smoke billowing out. Once the female officer retrieved the keys from our patient, the three cops were able to yank the man out of the vehicle (you know, because he decided to fight), and then they had to threaten to taze him because he was resisting arrest.

But wait, there's more!

The man did go to jail, but the woman in back was now homeless because she didn't have a key to Man 4's apartment-where her belongings were-and she couldn't stay with Man 1 because he lived with his sister, and Man 1's sister hates the patient because the patient apparently called child services on the sister for neglecting her children.

And that's not all.

Man 1 arrived about an hour after Man 4 was arrested and demanded we let him see the patient.

"Oh, are you her boyfriend?" I asked, pretending to know nothing at all.

He nodded and said frantically, "She texted me and said she was mugged. The guy stole the ring I just got her."

I bit my lip and sent Man 1 to the patient's room.

This started a fight because I guess a nurse went in the room to give the patient a hotline number to call regarding domestic violence and gave her advice to call the police station to see what she could do about getting her things out of Man 4's apartment, so Man 1 realized the patient lied and had still been seeing Man 4.

Not surprisingly in the least to any of us, the two quickly made up, and before the patient was released, her family, Man 1, and our patient were all posting huge, threatening rants on Facebook, tagging Man 4 in the status updates—as well as directly posting memes and threats on his Facebook wall.

But, you know what? Man 4 couldn't see the posts and still can't because when he made it to the pokey, the cops found out the man was wanted for felonies in three other states.

Meanwhile, the patient and Man 1 have broken up a few times, have been in a few more times for pregnancy tests, and I've seen the patient hanging all over two other men when I've seen her outside of my workplace.

Balls Deep

Okay, so if you don't think I'm a horrible person for the stories I've told so far, I may change your mind in a second.

A man came in with holes burned in the inner thighs of his jeans, and the crotch of his pants was bloody, as in the blood kept seeping into the fabric until it had no place to go but to the floor, where it made a huge mess. The man fell to his knees just as I jumped up to grab a wheelchair, and as he screamed in agony I rushed to the phone for help.

Nobody answered after a few rings, and I knew it was because they were getting ready for a Code Blue. Boy, shit was really hitting the fan.

Instead of running to the back like a fool and trying to find someone to come to the front, I did the only thing I could think of to grab the attention of everyone in back: I passed the patient in a life or death sprint, ran through the exit door, and hit the big button on the exterior pillar of the emergency room that sounds an alarm in the case of a severe trauma, chemical exposure, missing limb, or a patient cannot get inside without assistance.

Sure enough, hitting that button did the trick. Within seconds, several nurses rushed to the front, and all of them stopped in almost a shock-like state with expressions of confusion on their faces.

I was panting as I ran back inside, and now the patient was face-down and unconscious on the lobby floor.

"What happened to him?" one of the nurses asked me.

I quickly shut my mouth and tried to breathe through my nose to mask the fact that I desperately need to work out, and I'm pretty sure I almost passed out in the process because...well, I'm really out of shape and need to work out. (I sometimes start to work out, but this usually lasts about 10 seconds before I remember I have bacon in the fridge, and then I just get sidetracked...)

"What happened to him, Kerry?" the nurse repeated.

I shrugged and replied to him, "No idea. He just hobbled inside and fell on his knees."

"He didn't tell you what happened?"

"No," I said. "But he had blood all over the crotch of his jeans."

I motioned to the smudged trail on the floor. "A lot of blood."

Two nurses hurried to the back and returned with a stretcher. It took five adults to lift the man from the floor and situated him on a cot. He was then transported to a rauma room, and the doctor ordered that someone pop a smelling salts pill to wake the patient.

Now, I usually tell you I go to the back to drop off papers to the unit clerk, but in this case I went to the back just because I wanted to know what the hell was going on. It's really as simple as that.

I stood in the center of the nurses' station with the unit clerk as half of the nurses were still prepping in one room for the incoming code and the rest were trying to tend to the recently-woken patient. The doctor—the only doctor—we had that night did his best to help the RNs keep the patient under control, but this man came to losing his fucking mind. He was thrashing about violently and finally managed to bite the doctor.

Yep, doc was gonna be 'Patient Zero' for sure, and I was going to have to assemble my zombie apocalypse team.

The unit clerk stat paged security to the trauma room and it took 10 minutes to get the patient restrained. He still wasn't speaking besides repeating the word 'cunt' in the same tone back to back to back. I think we were all tired of the man's shouting and regretted bringing him to again.

"Tell me what happened," the charge nurse said to the patient for about the 14,000th time. She was losing her normally-calm demeanor and was starting to take deeper and longer inhalations.

Finally, the man spit out, "I blew up my balls. Help me. I blew up my balls."

Uh, hmm…

Is there an IC10 code for that?

"Thank you for calling Anthem BlueCross BlueShield. What is the patient's diagnosis?"

"Ma'am, the patient blew up his balls."

Anyway…

It took more prodding to hear from the man that he had been manufacturing meth in a two-liter soda bottle. In case you really need someone to tell you, don't try this at home because it's a really stupid fucking idea. I mean, making or using meth in general is stupid, but trying to make a portable lab so you don't blow up your double-wide is dumber than that.

"You burned yourself with meth?" the charge nurse asked, hoping to get the patient to confirm.

He was twitching and squirming as he replied that this was correct.

"Don't move," ordered the charge. She pushed gently on his shoulder and told him to stay still.

Our patient hollered like someone had just lynched him, and he then told the nurse not to touch him on the shoulder because it was sensitive from the car crash.

"When were you in a vehicular accident?" the doctor chimed in.

"Just now," the patient answered. "My bottle exploded and blew my balls off, and I wrecked. Oh my God. Can you save my balls? I can't live like a fixed dog. Please, save my balls."

Okay, okay, okay…Hold up. So, you're gonna make drugs that are <u>known to be prone to explosion</u> and you're going to stick the lab next to your most sensitive body parts as you're flying down a bumpy road?

Can't be sure or anything, but I'm not sure we thought this through.

"How about you try to do a few breathing exercises with Wanda over here while I take a quick peek at your injuries, okay?"

As soon as the doctor was able to cut off the front of the patient's jeans, he took a giant step back and exclaimed rather loudly, "Holy shit."

Of course, everyone in the room, the unit clerk, and I craned our necks in desperate attempts to see the patient's wounds.

'Holy shit' was an understatement.

I've seen men double over in pain and lose the ability to breathe for a few seconds after being kicked or hit in the testicular region, and though I have no way of confirming that it hurts so badly, I have assumed for most of my life that being whacked in the testicle is one of the worst pains a man can feel.

Well, you know what else probably hurts?

Answer: when your nutsack really has 'blown up,' leaving one testicle to hang down loosely under the tip of your dick and the other testicle to probably be rolling around on the baseboards of his busted-up car.

The patient's remaining testicle couldn't be saved, and while this story is probably not funny to some, I can't help but to feel amused when I think of it now. I understand drug abusers are not in the best frame of mind to make positive life choices, but the fact that this patient was dumb enough to place a meth lab contained only by plastic so thin I can squeeze the air out of the cavity and fold the plastic in half right next to his junk made me feel a little less compassionate for him.

<u>Play Ball</u>

In this next edition of 'how the hell did you think this was going to end, besides with you and your friends in the ER?', some of our patients were bringing back this old (possibly still-played?) sport called 'Slamball.'

If you're not familiar with Slamball, don't fret because I barely remembered it, either. I'm not much of a sports person (besides NHL—go Flyers), so I could be wrong when I tell you that Slamball seems to be pretty much like basketball with trampolines. Yeah. Trampolines.

When the players approach the net, they can jump on a set of trampolines affixed to the floor and surrounded by padding, and I guess the point is to hop on the trampoline to put you closer to the net and allow you to do things like twist in the air or do backflips or something before you try to put the ball in the net.

I have a few things to say about this.

Okay, so 1.) basketball already seems a little energy-consuming, with the running from end to end of the court and trying to make a basket, so I'm not sure if it was laziness that invented the trampolines by the nets or just someone trying to help a less-capable player to slam dunk. At any rate, and maybe it's because I work in the ER or I have seen a lot of those *America's Funniest Home Video* clips where people get feet stuck between the springs or fall to the ground in the middle of a flip, that makes me think this was a horrible idea.

So, 2.) aren't you already going pretty fast in basketball? If you refer to the first point, I mean, you're running, so it's not like you're slow-poking towards the net while you hold the ball under your arm and try to text your mom back about dinner with your weird uncle. Did we think that adding a trampoline was a good idea?

Obviously, someone was thinking more about the dunking aspect than the safety aspect of all of this, and I'm sure if I played basketball on a regular basis and didn't see 14-year-olds come in with their snapped-in-half bones protruding from their skin, I'd maybe think it was a fun idea to do this, too.

To get to the point I've been trying to make during all of this, Slamball was a sport performed by professional athletes. These people had their own teams and divisions and all of that. I thought the sport kind of fell off the grid around the mid-2000s, but I guess our patients decided to revive it…by setting up a bunch of those tiny exercise trampolines they had bought online or at garage sales at each end of a concrete basketball court. As if all those trampolines weren't enough, the group of men—fully grown, adult, old-enough-to-know-better, married with kids (most of them, anyway)—positioned a full-size trampoline in the center of the court. It was somehow low to the ground but capable of launching a player in the air, so what's better than a tool that leads to hundreds of injuries each year than one that's been modified and stripped of even the smallest safety features and installed incorrectly by a bunch of men looking to fly through the sky to dunk a ball in a net?

All of the trampolines were surrounded by pillows that were not fixed in place.

Can we all just close our eyes for one second and shake our heads a few times? I know I need to, and I bet you could use a break. Come on, do it. Let the confusion of why people do the things they do flow through you.

So, three men were brought to the hospital via some kind of big SUV by an uninjured teammate, and they all needed help getting out of the vehicle because they had another bright idea to put the middle seat down and lie next to one another in the back of the SUV to avoid the cost of the ambulance. One guy said he didn't care about the cost of an ambulance, but if his wife found out he was in one she would 'lose her shit' and he'd never hear the end of it.

Ugh.

What the fucking fuck.

Two of the men were wheeled to the lobby for registration because the RNs felt the men had not sustained injuries that required immediate medical intervention. And even though it was two in the morning…yes, I forgot to add it was fucking two in the morning when these men decided to do this…the waiting room was about a quarter filled. The wait times were about 20 to 30 minutes, so these men were registered like any other patients. I listed both of the chief complaints as falls, and one presented with the complaint that he thought his leg and arm were broken, while the other one clearly had a broken arm (his arm was basically twisted all the way around and was swollen), and he said he hit his head. <u>The man stressed his only complaint was his arm, despite having a headache</u>. Remember that. It's on the test.

The third injured member of the group was whisked away to the back, and I really couldn't tell where his nose was supposed to go because his face was covered with an ungodly amount of blood. He lost a tooth on the way to the back, and the driver of the SUV kind of kicked it around with the toe of his boot before picking it up, stuffing it in his pocket, and then asking me if I thought the dentist could put it back in the patient's mouth.

This is the point I learned what the guys were doing, so we're all caught up on the basics. But we never hear *just* the basics in the emergency room, do we?

Patient three hopped on the center court trampoline and tried to propel himself to the trampolines on one side of the court. This obviously went directly to plan because he ended up in the ER with his nose drooping down one of his cheeks.

I guess the man sustained his injuries when his leap wasn't as far as he thought it would be, meaning he fell face-first to the concrete court, a whopping six feet from the other set of trampolines. It was this patient's injuries that brought the group of friends to our hospital.

According to the driver, the other two men were on their respective trampolines by the net. One patient (the broken arm and leg guy) was trying to block his friend from making a basket, and he succeeded by shoving the second guy away from the net in mid-air. Man two missed the safety pillows and whacked the side of his head on the court, but he really felt the burn when he realized his arm had somehow landed under him…the man's palm was touching the small of his back while he was on the ground, and the patient told the driver that he couldn't feel his shoulder.

The men decided to actually prolong a trip to the ER until patient number three could try out his 'trick,' but when that trick fell flat (eek!), they packed it up for the night and decided it was time to visit us.

I know this story is bouncing around (damn, am I good with unintended puns or what?), but I feel it's best to kind of go out of order on this one to keep readers in the loop with everything that was happening.

The driver stayed at the desk and chatted, calling his friends dumbasses a few times and confirming the other three men had consumed copious amounts of alcohol.

When the head injury patient, without any warning at all, slumped and essentially slithered out of his wheelchair, the arm and leg patient yelled for help and the driver and I rushed to the waiting room to see exactly what was taking place.

"He was talking and just…I don't know," the arm and leg patient said. "He got this weird look in his eyes and then his eyes rolled back and he fell out of his chair. What the fuck is happening to him? Did he just pass out? Did the asshole just pass out on me, while I have broken bones?"

He then started hollering at the man, "Come on, prick. Get up and stop being a pussy."

"Don't move him," I ordered to the driver, who'd been in the process of rolling the patient over to face the waiting room ceiling.

"Wanda," I yelled, hoping the nurse was in triage.

I don't think she heard me, and other people in the waiting room had gathered around.

"Do something," one of the women waiting screamed at me. "Do CPR or something. Don't you have to shock him now, you know with the paddles?"

Several of the onlookers appeared to grow excited by this woman's suggestions, and it occurred to me that they didn't really care about the wellbeing of the patient passed out on the floor. They cared about the action.

They cared about whipping out their cell phones and taking pictures like a few of them were doing. They cared about being able to jump on Facebook and post a status update like, 'OMFG. Totes just saw dude about 2 die && then DR said clear & shocked him back 2 lyfe. LOL.'

"Wanda!" I screamed again, to the point that the lower portion of my throat stung. "I need you now."

She heard me that time, and Wanda came running from the triage room with her Littman stethoscope whacking her chest and her navy clogs a-clappin' on the tile lobby floor.

"Did he just fall out of his chair?" she asked the man's friend, as she tried to gather information.

"He had a head injury," I told her. "But he said it wasn't bad, and they told me to register him and send him to triage."

"Tell me what happened to bring this man here," Wanda instructed of the other wheelchair-bound patient and the driver.

She recognized the gleams in their eyes and speedily added, "Short version. Tell me about the injury."

Both men started talking at once and Wanda was growing frustrated.

"Driver said the other guy knocked him out of the air, patient hit the side of his head on the ground, and landed on his arm."

"Yeah," said the driver. "That. That's what happened."

"Hey," said the other patient. "Don't blame this shit on me. Ya'll were okay with it. And I'm not going around blaming you fuckers for my fucked up leg."

He groaned and tried to hold up his arm.

"You know what?" he slurred. "Fuck all ya'll. Tryin' to take me to court and bullshit over this asshole not being able to sit up straight."

I realized we were all quiet and staring at the patient with confused expressions on our faces.

Wanda snapped out of it and ordered me to call the back for assistance. This man needed to go to the back immediately, meaning some of the patients in back were going to have to be doing a little bit of moving around.

As I was halfway to the desk to call for help, Wanda shrieked at me in a tone I hadn't heard from her before or since, "Kerry, tell them he needs a trauma room right now. Call a code. Call a code right now."

I hurried to the phone and wasn't sure if I needed to call the code first or call the back. I was caught up in the pressure of new patients and visitors coming through the front door, could hear the commotion of all the people in the waiting room, heard Wanda's panicky voice repeating in my head as well as her yelling at bystanders to step back, and I freaked out.

"Kerry," Wanda yelled to me, noticing by looking through the waiting room window to the registration desk that I was frozen with a look of utter fear. "Kerry, call the back. Okay? Call the back. Call charge. Then hang up and call a code. Come on. I need you to do this right now. We need this man in a room right now."

My hands were shaking as I tried to dial the charge nurse, and just like in my repetitive nightmares, I dialed the wrong number three times before I finally hit the correct combination of digits.

As the phone was ringing, I was trying to figure out why I was trembling. Why then? I made it through patient suicide attempts just fine. I made it through registering infants we all knew were close to death. Blood and bones and seizures came through that entrance on a daily basis, and I was the calm one. I was always the calm one when it came to that kind of stuff, and my 'freaking out' in the past simply involved hurrying to notify a certified responder. It was never anything like I was experiencing then. I realized I stopped breathing and gasped for air just as someone answered.

"Yeah?"

"Wanda needs a trauma room ASAP and I'm calling a code. Send help."

The charge nurse was in the middle of trying to ask me a question, but it was almost like I had no control of hanging up on her. My brain didn't feel like it was sending messages to my hands; they were acting on their own, and my thoughts were ricocheting between feeling guilty for hanging up on the nurse versus knowing I needed to call the code for the patient.

"Kerry," Wanda asked, "did you call?"

"Yes," I yelled. "They're coming."

"Good. Now call the code. This gentleman's friend is going to calmly step outside and call the patient's wife. He's going to tell her that we need her here as soon as she can get here safely."

She always had a way with that, with knowing when to speak directly or indirectly to someone, with knowing how to sound authoritative but sweet, with knowing how to keep us all steady but efficient.

I watched the driver go outside as I picked up the phone again and called the code.

"Are you even going to look at me?" I heard a woman say.

And then I did. I raised my glance to a woman holding a fast food bag and a large drink.

"I said I need to get back to my friend's room," she said.

"It's going to be a minute before I can get security," I said in a rush.

She shook her head. "This is bullshit."

She took a look around, saw the old man hacking blood in a hanky behind her, saw the crowd in the waiting room, saw the stretcher coming out between the double doors to the left of us.

"You should have someone out here for this."

That was her reaction to everything going on around her. For all I knew, there was a man who could have been dying in the waiting room, and I was going to have to bench three more patients—two of whom looked genuinely ill.

But no. No, was this witch worried about any of that? Not even a little bit. She was more concerned with making sure she got upstairs before her fries were anything but piping hot.

"I need you to sit down, and I'll call security for you."

The woman switched her soda from one hand to the other and used her now-free hand to swipe the signs and pens and clipboard that were on the countertop to the lobby floor.

"Fuck you," she said. "I'm not sitting down. I was here first and all of these people are going to wait until I'm helped."

The nurses from the back had lifted the waiting room patient to the stretcher, and as they were headed back to the ER I saw small creeks of pinkish watery blood trickling from the patient's ears, and there was an alarming amount of vermillion blood steadily streaming from the man's nostrils. His eyes were open, but they were half-rolled back. His mouth was partially agape, and I watched for his chest to rise and fall, but that only happened once in the time it took for the nurses to wheel him to the back.

Wicked old witch of the front desk saw the patient but wasn't at all moved.

I wasn't arguing with her then and I had no intentions of doing so. I called the code for the patient and instead of hanging up the phone, I asked the operator to do something else for me: stat page security to escort a visitor from the property.

This probably wasn't the smoothest move, you know, and I usually don't try to further instigate trouble, but I was in no mood to deal with the woman, especially after she had knocked all of my stuff to the floor, meaning not only would I have to stop to pick it all up, but I'd have to sanitize everything with cleaner that had a two-minute wet time. Two minutes of waiting while your husband's hanky is filling up with blood because he can't stop coughing is practically a lifetime. Damn this bitch for screwing with my job and my routine.

She didn't seem angry, though, when I told the operator I needed security for a visitor escort. Instead, she laughed and called me a bunch of names that made the lady behind her gasp.

I just shook my head and waited for backup because there was no way in holy hell I was going around that counter to pick up my clipboard with even the slightest fear that the woman was going to kick me in the head while I was hunched over.

Someone called to the front and told me to start moving patients around on the tracking board. I was supposed to shift all of the patients in trauma rooms to the right, meaning one of the patients was either already moved to another unit to continue the examination, or that patient was on the way. This doesn't happen unless we're completely full and a real emergency comes in.

And as if I didn't recognize that we were in the middle of a real emergency, the charge nurse made sure to let me know for sure by locking down the back. Nobody in. Nobody out. All available nurses were to be helping with the patient requiring the most attention, and I knew it was the man they'd just rushed to the back. There were going to be no discharges during the lockdown. The waiting room wait time was about to be doubled, at least, and sorry 'bout 'cha if you wanted to go back to see your friend's brother's aunt who came in because her dog stepped on her foot. The rules were strict. The rules were simple. Nobody goes in. Nobody comes out. Patients are to stay in their rooms. This keeps the halls clear for our ER RNs and docs, as well as allows other departments to head down to the patient's room without having to worry about meeting a bed in the hall on another patient's way to CT.

Wanda came running out from the back part and was looking around.

"Where's the driver?"

I nodded toward the door. "Still on the phone, I think."

She hurried outside and I could see her talking to the man. I think a family member would view her as calm, but I knew from the way she was rapidly moving her hands as her mouth moved that something was very wrong. She was trying to stress the importance of the patient's family arriving without saying the words: this man could die.

Well, shit.

Have you ever stopped right in the midst of chaos to appreciate something that seems silly, like the clarity of the sky or the 65-degree-temperature or the smell of a sweet perfume in the air?

I did that in that moment. Everything around me screeched to a halt. There was no chatter from the waiting room. The hanky man and his wife were frozen in time. Miss

Priss at the front desk was in the middle of slurping her Diet Mt. Dew. I couldn't hear the phones, and the lights of another approaching ambulance were stopped in the middle of a rotation.

The only thing I could notice was how beautiful the sky looked from what I could see on the security monitors. It was a blanket of navy swirled with black, gently caressing speckles of white. Right there in the center was half a moon, a cookie cutter version of the silhouette of the Mr. Moon toys I had from McDonald's when I was a child. On a night when the sky looked like that, there wasn't supposed to be such chaos taking place around me.

Yet, in a split second, it all picked up again and the noise was deafening.

Security was on the line when I answered the phone.

"We're up here with the addict from last night," the guard said. "He's fighting. We need you to walk people up."

"I need help making someone leave," I said.

"Tell them to leave," the guard instructed. "If that doesn't work, call the cops. We're too busy to come down there. Sorry."

I frequently use the phrase 'fuck my life,' and it's almost always used while I'm on the clock because, well, you've read the books.

I hung up the phone and looked to the woman at the desk. She was tapping her fingers on the empty countertop and was huffing loudly.

"Well?" she asked.

"I'm going to have to ask you to leave the property for the night," I said sternly.

She started throwing her fit. She stomped around and screamed and threatened me and then started threatening other patients if they approached the desk.

This is when I called the cops.

Right around the time the police arrived, so did the head injury patient's wife. Also around this time, I was finally able to call the hanky man to the desk to register, and I had already fielded about 20 'when will I be seen's from the waiting room crowd.

While the cops were talking to the woman from the front desk, I notified the charge nurse that the wife for the trauma patient was up front, and that woman waited patiently while I registered the hanky guy. I didn't think she looked like anything was wrong. If I didn't know any better, I would guess she was there to visit someone on the floor.

"What'd the idiot do now?" she asked me. "He's always doing something."

She didn't know.

"Um," I said, "he fell. A nurse is coming up for you now, and she'll tell you more."

The woman laughed. "He fell? That's all?"

A nurse did come out, but she walked to the patient's wife with the house supervisor at her side.

"Your husband hit his head and fractured his skull," I heard the supervisor telling the woman from registration's little office located behind the front desk.

"How bad is it?" the wife asked.

There was a pause.

"There's a lot of pressure on his brain right now."

"What does that mean?"

The nursing supervisor took over and said, "Part of his brain is being crushed right now, basically."

The patient's wife broke down and the woman from the front desk was getting loud because for some unknown reason, she was being handcuffed.

The patient in the back was transferred via helicopter to another hospital for surgery to alleviate the pressure on his brain, and the woman from the front desk was arrested for possession of meth. Shocker there.

Our Slamball participant survived his surgery, but he's now living in an assisted living facility. His other friends were discharged and went home to their families. We've heard rumors that the families have been threatening to sue each other, but I honestly hope it doesn't come to that.

__Things We Sometimes Want to Say to Patients__

-Did you seriously just ask me what the difference was between *ammonia* and *pneumonia*?

-So, let me get this straight...You can sit in the waiting room for an hour and a half, and you can wait as long as it takes for someone to come by your room with Dilaudid, yet you want the medi-cab waiting for you the very second you get discharged because you got what you want and now are ready to go home?

-Dude, the Dollar Tree sells soap *and* deodorant. So no, I'm not resting my face against my propped-up palm; I'm trying to keep the sleeve of my shirt over my nostrils so I don't gag and aspirate on my puke.

-You're fucking with me, right? Tell me you can't possibly be this stupid.

-Sign in, sit down, and shut up. Don't come to the desk 900 times and stare at me until I finally make eye contact, which you find as your cue to ask, "How much longer?"

-You called 911 for that?!

-You drove here at two in the morning during a blizzard for that?!

-You were just a dick to me for no good reason. In return, I just told the nurse that you seem to appear and be acting like any average healthy person, so maybe they should take the five or six patients behind you in line to rooms first.

-Holy shit, you've been here 38 times this month. Why don't you ask if you can just buy a room? You're practically already living here.

-Calling your nurse a whore is a pretty stupid idea when you start to think that she's going to pick the gauge of the needle used to give you that pain medication…you know, when she has time to give it to you.

-Well, that sure was a stupid fucking idea, huh? Bet you won't be doing that again.

-How the hell did you make it this far in life?

-Go home, take some Ibuprofen, and go the fuck to sleep. Stop clogging up our rooms with your bullshit attempts to get attention.

-Some families go on vacation to destinations such as Disneyland. And then some families go vacation to the ER. I think we'll make some shirts that say, 'I went to the ER and all I got was this shirt that covers my side boob and the belly that hangs over my thighs.'

<u>Fucking Seriously?</u>

Right in the middle of three hours of sleep, my Facebook messenger started pinging like mad and my phone was ringing off the hook.

I don't like being woken up that way unless there's an emergency or I don't have to go to work, but of course, I couldn't be so lucky. Apparently a co-worker had called in, leaving one person to work an evening shift— which is probably possible to accomplish when hell freezes over, but not so much otherwise. So our supervisor was coming in to 'work' with that coworker until relief could be found.

The problem in this was our supervisor knows nothing about our computer software. Nothing. He can't register patients. He can't transfer rooms. He can't discharge. He doesn't know how to scan insurance cards or even enter the information in the system if my coworker had been the one gathering the information for data entry. Essentially, this supervisor was and is useless on any shift. I guess 'if your job is to tell me how to do my job, you need to know how to do my job' is accurate here, right?

Anyway, I stupidly agreed to come in because I figured I could use the overtime to pay down some debt. I got up, made a milkshake, and took a ham and cheese Lunchable (dinner of champions for a 13-hour shift, right?) from the fridge before I headed to work.

Wow. What a damn disaster I walked into when I got to work.

My coworker was sweating profusely and the desk was layered with paperwork. The phone was ringing non-stop. People waiting to be seen were backed up to the door, and the waiting room was full. I took a quick glance at the tracking board. Five of the 12 ungreened patients (information hasn't been gathered—green means they're good to discharge) in the back were being discharged and nobody had gotten their information, meaning if everything wasn't up to date, the hospital was going to have one hell of a time getting paid. In turn, that would come back on us and someone would tell us we weren't doing our jobs correctly. Shit rolls downhill, you know. I couldn't even see where the bottom of the tracking board was. Wait times were pushing four hours, and some of this was registration's fault because the nurses had to choose between waiting for someone to gather patient information versus releasing the patient and hoping everything was okay.

Meanwhile, while I was in the process of clocking in and my coworker was trying not to have a panic attack, our supervisor stood with his back against a wall and his hands folded neatly over his abdomen. He was doing nothing but watching the crowds grow and watching my coworker freak out.

"We're so backed up right now," my coworker frantically told me. "I can't do this."

I put my milkshake on the desk and started digging in to all the work. All the while, our boss continued to do absolutely nothing. (There's kind of a point to this, but I'm going to be honest and say I'm mostly using it for reiteration that we were really freaking busy.) It took my coworker and I—two very competent workers—more than an hour to get caught up.

"Well," said our supervisor, "I'm going to go home, unless you want me to stick around to help you more."

And in the moment I almost got fired, I spouted off, "And just have you been helping us?"

I think my saving grace during this time was a pissed off frequent flyer who came to the desk with his daughter.

"My dad's been waiting for two hours," the daughter shouted. "His back is killing him. You call this an emergency room? What would happen if he came in with his arm chopped off? Would he still be sitting in the waiting room?"

I wanted to tell her no, that if her dad came in with a missing limb it really would be an emergency, and he'd be taken straight back.

But, *since my supervisor was there* and I strive to offer *superior customer service*, I introduced the patient's daughter to my boss and told her this was an opportunity for her to voice her opinions to someone in charge.

My supervisor handled the situation quite well (this is why we need a sarcasm font) by bluntly stating to the patient and his daughter, "Your back can't be hurting that bad. Go back to your seats and someone will eventually get to you."

Ha ha.

I laughed inside then and laugh now because I knew what was coming.

See, I've dealt with this patient's daughter about 9000 times. I know that smiling, telling her you'll notify the triage nurse, and then offering her a cup of instant decaf coffee that tastes like it was brewed in 1987 will calm her down and we won't see her at the desk again until someone calls for her father. I know that any other response sets this woman off to the point that security has to be notified. And I could have informed my supervisor of this, but why let him miss out on a learning experience?

The patient's daughter ripped off her ball cap and stepped forward, almost to the point that she was leaning over our counter.

"And just who the fuck are you, you low-life piece of dog shit?"

Verbatim. Like, I've thought about ordering a sign with these words and giving it to my boss for the next holiday.

Making matters even worse, our supervisor laughed in this woman's face and informed her of some long, official title that could have been summed up by 'this department's director,' but I suspect the supervisor was feeling on top of the totem pole and didn't feel there were repercussions for the kind of behavior that would send me packing in two-seconds flat.

Never one to back down from a confrontation, the patient's daughter gripped the bill of her ball cap, stretched over the desk as far as she could reach, and tried to hit our supervisor with the hat.

"Lady, what is your problem?" he asked her.

As the woman started to walk around the desk to get her hands on the supervisor, she shrieked, "You're my problem, asshole. Coming in here, thinking you know it all, thinking you're better than everyone with your flaky pube mustache."

I picked up the phone to call security, and quickly said to my supervisor, "Welcome to ER registration."

He hurried to the restroom and locked himself inside until security calmed the woman down and told her to sit in the waiting room with her pained father. Security then had to escort our supervisor across the building at the man's request.

Well, if that wasn't just a load of fun!

With the almost-fight behind us and patients still flooding in, I noticed my polo was spotted in sweat.

As I was talking to ICU on the phone and had the phone cord stretched across the room so I could continue the paperwork for a newly-registered patient, a teenager rushed to the center of the lobby and let out a scream you hear in horror movies.

"Let me call you back," I said to the woman from ICU. I hung up the phone and kind of offered the teenager a blank stare, hoping she'd just tell me what was wrong instead of dramatically expecting someone to run to her with cuddles.

She clenched her fists and lifted her arms in front of her chest like you see people doing in movies when they're sobbing and begging.

"He's dying!" she shrieked.

Damn. This girl needed to be on the stage or something, for all the attention she was gathering.

"Tell me what's going on," I said, unamused.

She pointed to a car parked just outside the entrance. I saw three young men pulling another man out of the backseat, and then one of the three stepped back and vomited.

"Tell me what's going on right now," I sternly said to the blubbering girl.

She whipped around and extended her arms to show me her wrists and said, "He sliced them. Oh, there was so much blood."

I turned to get the triage nurse from the back as everyone looked on, but I then came to my senses and asked, "Wait. Is he still bleeding?"

The girl shook her head and said, "Well, no. He wrapped his wrists up because it wasn't killing him."

Holy fucking crap. I wasn't about to rush this kid to the back just because he was probably seeking attention. I know it sounds horrible, but we see this all the time. Someone (and I know it's a HUGE stereotype, but they're usually in the 15-25 age range) will come in saying they 'overdosed' and get rushed to a trauma room in the middle of our rush hour, but then the truth will come out that the patient's version of overdosing means he or she took five Tylenol instead of two.

"And he took a bunch of pills," the teenager said to me. "Like, he took a bottle of his grandma's pain killers and then a bottle of Oxy. I think he took blood thinner."

"Shit," I mumbled. "Wanda, we need you out here for a suicide attempt."

Now, all these bystanders were perfectly fine with watching the show, but when they became part of it by hearing someone was going to the back before they were, it pissed them off. While I was trying to register this teenager for his suicide attempt from information gathered by four other teenagers, people from the waiting room kept interrupting and cutting in line, demanding to be taken to the back.

I mostly tried to ignore these people and continue with registration, which took about 10 minutes longer than usual because nobody would leave me alone long enough to get it done.

The triage nurse found two nurses passing through from OB to assist her in removing the suicide attempt from the vehicle out front and transfer the kid to a stretcher. He was unconscious when he was wheeled through, and seeing how badly the patient needed immediate medical intervention calmed some of the nagging patients, but others continued to bitch and moan.

"Call his parents," I ordered the kids at the desk.

One of his friends shook his head and said, "Nope. He's emancipated from them but was homeless, so he moved in to the apartment above his grandma's house."

I think my eyes almost popped out of my head when I said, "So? Call his grandma, then."

"Can't. She died like two months ago."

"What the fuck?" I asked, doing little to hide my confusion, surprise, and frustration. "Does he have any family to notify?"

Miss Emmy Nominee chimed in that she was the patient's girlfriend and had been dating him for a month, so that automatically made her the closest person to a relative that he had.

That's not how this works. That's not how any of this works.

All four of the teens decided on their own that they were going back to the patient's room, but my coworker and I teamed up to nix that.

"You bitches can't keep me from my boyfriend," scoffed the drama queen.

I shook my head and let my coworker explain exactly to the teen just what rights she had to the patient at the moment and that the four friends needed to sit down until a nurse came out for them. The kids made a few smartass remarks but complied.

The patient in back wasn't unconscious for long, and we realized he was conscious when we heard a male scream out shrilly, "Get the fuck away from me you skanky motherfucking whore!"

Hey, I recognized that voice.

Of course! How could I not have noticed?

The teen in the back had been admitted to the hospital just a few months earlier, also for a suicide attempt. Back then, I guess, he tried to shoot himself in the head, but he didn't have the strength to hold the gun steady, so the bullet grazed the patient's scalp and he had to get the wound glued.

There's a shit-ton more to this story.

It turns out the patient took video footage of every one of his suicide attempts—from the gunshot wound to the wrist-slicing to the pills—and this was discovered by another friend.

"I need help right now," a young man said to me, as he wiped tears from his eyes.

Bear with me.

"What's the problem today?"

I thought he was going to need a mental health eval, and that was not going to be a good thing with the board as full as it was. I hate, hate, hate having to bench a mental health patient during a long waiting time. I swear, I always get goosebumps when I see these people get tired of waiting and walk out the door; I'm always afraid I'll next see them in the obituary section of the newspaper.

Someone recently questioned a previous story where a mental health patient repeatedly came in for help and made threats but was sent home instead of transferred, but when we're busy or the other hospital is busy and full, or when the patient has already BEEN to those facilities and is non-compliant in treatment, there's no place for these people to go, and they usually get in trouble when they leave. I may not know all the lingo for what it's called when someone's vital signs fall off the grid and their heart stops beating while they're dead on the hallway floor or when a woman's heart monitor falls to zero and an alarm goes off or exactly how a procedure is performed, but I know I work at this job sometimes 18-days in a row, and with this part, especially, I kind of have a small idea of what goes on. Nobody said it was right. Nobody said this is how it works in big cities or places that have their shit together. But this is how it works HERE.

"My friend just tried to kill himself."

I hadn't put two and two together yet.

"Um, okay. Is he here right now?"

I meant in a car or something, so when the guy in front of me responded, "Yes," I took a deep breath, told him to wait, and headed for triage.

"Fucking seriously?" we both said at the same time when I told Wanda we had another suicide attempt.

"No," the guy at the desk called to us. "He's your patient right now. I need help because I found a bunch of stuff I need you to take care of."

"What?" I asked, so lost.

Now THIS is when the young man explained he discovered the patient had not only recorded his suicide attempts, but he had also uploaded them to the internet and shared them to a special thread in a community of users with self-harm fetishes. The patient's friend apparently found evidence that the patient had found an online friend, shared details about his life, and then said he wanted to kill himself. Well, the online 'friend' encouraged the patient to do so, and then we were right where we were, listening to this patient go nuts.

During the patient's ER visit, he spit on all of our security guards, urinated on a nurse, bit through his IV line, and he punched a doctor.

In the end, the patient was admitted as a critical case due to his overdose, and then he was an ED to mental health because one of the mental health officers took the patient's records to a judge and the judge agreed with mental health that the patient needed to be admitted for his own protection…protection from himself.

<u>Elephant in the Room</u>

Let's talk about something a lot of people know happens, but is often left unspoken: the treatment of medical professionals.

Now, I can definitely understand how ETOH patients and drug users can present combative against staff. Though I can't excuse their behavior, these patients are not in the clearest frame of mind. They may know the difference between right and wrong, but there's something there leaving these people with impaired judgement. I've never decked someone while I've been drinking, but I've sure had my fair share of falling all over the place and drunk dialing after one too many shots of tequila.

No. Let's talk about the violence that everyone turns their heads from. Let's talk about a 350-pound man grabbing the wrist of a 125-pound nurse and throwing her up against the wall because he wants pain medication and he wants it now. Let's talk about how patients come in and leave nurses with black eyes or swollen cheeks or bruises on their arms because the patients were simply unsatisfied.

It seems a large portion of society seems to have the attitude that because someone 'signed up' for a medically-positioned job that this employee is therefore supposed to 'expect' and tolerate abuse, whether it be verbal or physical.

On a regular basis, techs, RNs, CNAs, doctors, and other hospital staff in reach of patients are kicked, spit on, bitten, punched, groped, and hit. These incidents are not isolated to our hospital, but when a healthcare professional is in a violent situation, he or she may feel alone because there seems to be a thin line of support for these victims. And, unfortunately, unless the attacks are severe enough to result in death or injuries such as broken bones, they are largely ignored by law enforcement or administration because these bouts of assault are considered to be occupational hazards.

People, it's time to wake the hell up. It's really as simple as that.

I hate going to Wal Mart, where they have 24 checkout lines, yet only two are open and the wait time is a good 30 minutes before I can even start unloading the items in my cart, but I can't get away with popping my cashier in the nose simply because I was sick of waiting.

I can't go to Burger King and slam the cook's head against the counter because I was hungry and didn't get my burger in the minute and a half I thought I should have it.

If we are expected to remain civilized in public, during times we are surrounded by stress and frustration and have our kids crying because they wanted a candy bar and mom said no, then we should expect civility from patients. Healthcare workers understand the stress patients undergo when registering to the ER, and we all try to see the situation from families' points of view throughout the hospital visit. I can tell you with most certainty that a nurse will be far more likely to forgive an 86-year-old Alzheimer's patient for waking up in fear and shoving her aside than when a 26-year-old woman clocks her in the cheek because the nurse had to relay to the patient that the doctor refused to refill a narcotic prescription.

We need to support our hospital staff, and this needs to happen now—not when you see another nurse covered in bruises, not when you see the news report of a doctor shot in his back as he was walking to a car, not when you hear the housekeeper was jumped by someone desperate for keys to the pharmacy. We need to wake up and realize that we all deserve to feel safe at our jobs. Nobody needs to wake up and wonder if this is the night some disgruntled patient is going to return and shoot everyone.

Support hospital staff and discourage violence against our nation's healthcare workers.

A few years ago this man was mad because I told him he wasn't supposed to drink or eat until he was seen by a doctor, so he threw the contents of his Big Gulp on me and called me a 'cunt muffin.'

All this time later, I'm still wondering what that even is. I'm afraid to Google it.

<u>Whew-ee!</u>

You never know exactly what kind of patient you're gonna get when he or she comes in and has been participating in illegal drug usage.

Most of the time, though, you can pretty much bet that the drug-using patient is going to be a huge pain in the ass because when you pump yourself full of battery acid and anhydrous ammonia, it's like you gain super strength and lose inhibition.

One night we heard the radio beep, followed by a dispatcher assigning a medic to a violent middle-age woman diagnosed with a bouquet of illnesses from the mental illnesses garden…who'd admitted to taking bath salts.

Great. That's just fucking great. I wasn't upset that I was going to have to actually do something on this slow night; I was upset because the dispatcher said the patient was violent, and that's before she was in an 8x10 glass room with people ordering her around.

When the patient arrived to the hospital, it was a pain in the ass to get her to comply with any sort of direction. The woman refused to sit on the cot. She refused to undress. Then when she finally undressed, she refused to put on a gown. She refused to stay in her room. She refused to keep her voice down.

Basically, she was just walking around the back part of the ER naked until security could get down there, and then she was pacing the corners of her room naked and screaming after that.

"There are bugs in my heart," she screamed so loudly I could hear her words crystal clear from the registration area. "I feel them eating my arteries. I'm going to have a heart attack because these bugs are eating me alive."

"Ma'am," I guess the doctor said, "we see no evidence of bugs on you."

"They're living in my pussy," the woman screamed back. "I have a colony of bugs in my pussy."

This went on and on for about an hour. Security had to fight with the patient several times to keep her in the room. She tried three times to act innocent, but then run full-speed by the officers, but I guess you think you're running faster than you really are when you're high on a drug that includes Sudafed in the recipe section.

"Oh," she screamed. "The bugs have invaded my pussy. They're in my tits. They're in my heart. Someone help me; I'm being invaded by bugs."

The doctor ordered a urine specimen from the patient, but this woman refused that, too. She said she just wanted to be able to create one of those 'fund me' websites by going to the hospital so she could ask people to pay her medical bills, but said she really wanted the money to go toward, uh, recreational substances. She started spitting, kicking, and screaming that she just wanted the bugs out of her vagina and out of her heart.

In order to get a urine specimen from the patient, a tech lied to her by saying we couldn't get the bugs out of her vaginal area unless we could test them to find out which medicine would kill them off. The woman agreed to give a sample, and as soon as she put that half-filled cup in the little specimen window, our tech took the urine and literally ran across the ER to avoid having to deal with the patient any further.

There wasn't much our doctors could do for the woman, from what I was told, to get the drugs out of her system. It was a long game of 'wait and see.' During this time, the patient cried and hit the glass wall of her room, angry because she was duped into peeing in a cup. (The urine sample, by the way, showed the patient had mixed her bath salts with a lovely bunch of cocaine.)

The patient was (finally!) restrained shortly after hitting the glass, when she tried to tear her left breast open by scratching repeatedly at her skin.

The patient was admitted to mental health to detox, and then we learned she went to jail upon her discharge date because she pulled down her pants in the parking lot and peed on a bush.

When the Mood Strikes

We had a pretty unique incident happen a few years back.

Now, it's not all that unusual that a husband and wife are placed in the same nursing home. It's also not completely unheard of that both husband and wife will end up in our ER at the same time for injuries or illnesses.

But what took place is kind of, uh, a special occurrence…to our ER, at least.

A nurse walked in a non-trauma room to administer a dose of pain medication but wasn't in there long.

"Did someone take my patient to the bathroom?" she asked to a relatively slow nurses' station.

Nobody answered, so she clapped her hands to get everyone's attention. "Hey," she yelled. "Did someone take my guy in eight to the bathroom?"

This time, she heard a bunch of scattered, "No,"s or, "I didn't"s, and these answers really set her off because she then announced her patient—a man in his late 90s—was missing from his room. To make matters worse, the man had dementia and often wandered out of his room at the nursing home. It became so bad at the nursing home that a CNA had to be stationed right outside his door on a regular basis to steer him back to his bed at night.

"Kerry," she said to me, wiggling her index finger.

"No, no, no," I laughed. "If I'm back here I have to watch the monitors. I have to be able to see if people are coming in."

"Wanda will watch the front," she said. "I need you to walk around out front and make sure this guy isn't in the parking lot or something. And if he isn't there, check around the waiting room and the bathrooms. I'm gonna check the back. How does this kind of stuff always happen to me?"

I wondered the same thing, how I always managed to be around so many crazy incidents that I was able to churn them out dozens at a time in a book with multiple editions. Nuts, right? (I've come to the conclusion that a higher power has placed me in this position for this very purpose.)

Well, while Wanda was taking my place at the desk, I went outside and looked up and down every row in the dimly-lit parking lot. I saw three stray cats, two skunks, and a whole lot of trash, but the elderly man wasn't anywhere around as far as I could see. And when I went back inside and checked the waiting room and the bathrooms, the man wasn't there, either.

"Where the hell is he?" the nurse asked, more to the universe than to me. Her eyes filled with tears and her hands were starting to shake. And her fear was completely understandable. I mean, I don't know anyone who's ever lost a patient at this job, really, but I can't imagine that the outcome would be all that great.

"I'm going to lose my job," she panicked. "I'm going to be homeless. Oh my god. I'm gonna have to give blowjobs to random men."

My facial expression directly following that statement can be described as the following: my eyes were kind of wide in the moment, with my gaze fixed on the nurse. My mouth was partially hanging open and for so long that my lips were drying out.

"Uh…I don't think it's going to come to that," I said with an awkward 'huh-huh-huh' laugh.

That sure escalated quickly, didn't it? How the hell did we get from a missing man to the nurse being homeless and giving blowjobs?

Phew.

A woman from lab entered the ER from the back way and noticed the nurse by my side was now full-blown crying—I mean this woman had snot bubbles exploding out of her nostrils and her eyeliner was running down her cheeks and she was seriously freaking the fuck out. So, doing what I would do in this situation, the lab lady made a face that said 'nope, not touching that one' and she walked the long way to get to her patient's room.

I tried to comfort the nurse, but I'm about good at this task as a walrus is at crossing a tightrope. I never know the right things to say, laughter is my nervous response, and even when I'm sincere, the words don't come out sounding that way. Most of the time, if I'm going to offer comfort in any way, it's going to be of the Southern kind, and it's going to come to you in a brown paper bag. Judge all you want, but I do what I can and excel at what I can do.

The lab worker screamed in shock, staggered back, and took the trauma room's curtain with her as she bumped into the countertop of the nurses' station.

She stammered, "Uh, uh. I need some help. From anyone."

I definitely wasn't going to volunteer to go down there, just in case the floor was covered by vomit, but I was comfortable standing and watching as three nurses hurried to the trauma room.

Two of these nurses gasped, and the third one…He started laughing and couldn't stop. Tears were falling down his cheeks and his breaths became wheezes in a matter of seconds.

The nurse at my side grew annoyed just as quickly.

"Yep," she said with a growl. "It's always fun and games to everyone around here."

One of the two shocked nurses from down the hall called to my anxiety-riddled nurse, "Found your patient."

The woman gave a smirk and a wink, and that's when I knew I had to walk that way.

As the frantic nurse and I neared the room, I could hear faint moans.

"Is that what it sounds like?" I whispered.

The nurse walking with me shook her head. "Can't be."

Oh, but it sure was.

Our nurse's missing patient was the trauma room patient's husband.

And they were doin' the dirty right there in that woman's bed, despite her being in the ER in the first place for a fall.

The patients continued their business, even with the curtain missing and people standing just outside the room, as if nothing else meant much or even existed, for that matter.

Some of the nurses deliberated on what to do, but they finally settled on two of them taking each side of the curtain and holding it taut across the room's entrance and glass windows.

I guess the patient and his wife were, ahem, unoccupied a few minutes later and the man tried to sneak back to his room but was surprised to see the nurses waiting for him outside his wife's room.

When asked about the incident by the doctor, the husband replied, "They don't let me fuck my wife anymore."

The doctor had to leave the room because he couldn't stop laughing.

As it turns out, the patient stated the nursing home banned its residents from engaging in intercourse and separated the two because they kept sneaking out of their rooms at night to fornicate. Our patient stated most of his falls were sustained on his way to his wife's room, and she said most of her falls were sustained in the same fashion, including the fall that put her in the hospital on the night in question.

To my knowledge, the nursing home kept the couple separated because "policies are policies."

One of my favorite RNs ever came up to me with an expression of confusion mixed with disgust.

"What's up?" I asked.

"Did you hear that patient in triage?"

I shook my head.

"I asked the patient if she lives with family and she said yes, that the man with her was her boyfriend."

"Okay," I shrugged. "What's weird about that?"

"She then said the man is also her cousin. I told her I didn't know what to say, and she said they get that reaction a lot."

Registration's Falling Down, Falling Down, Falling Down...

A mother and father rushed inside and pushed through the crowded lobby until they stood at the desk. I was about to inform the two that we could only have one family at the desk at a time, but I took a quick look at dad's outstretched arms and knew someone needed to take the couple straight back.

"Wanda," I called, while trying to keep my tone relatively steady as to not cause panic to the crying parents or other people in the lobby.

And then my brand-new, three-days-on-the-job, 'I can handle anything; don't worry'-coworker stood up, saw the little boy dangling in dad's arms, and said loudly, "Holy fuck. Someone get some help right now!"

I closed my eyes and shook my head.

Wanda walked around the corner from triage and saw what we saw: a pre-teen child with missing teeth, bloody foam oozing out of his mouth, an eye so swollen it was probably the size of a golf ball (if not larger), lacerations to his cheeks, patches of missing hair, scraped knees, torn clothing, and an ear that somehow had been ripped from just above the boy's lobe to the inner ear.

Though the child was unconscious, my coworker was not. She had taken to shoving the sleeve of her sweater in her mouth, biting down, and making these weird concerned noises like, "Ee! Ooh!"

I shot her a look, but her eyes were clenched tight and she was rocking to her left and right while she chewed on her shirt.

Wanda hurried the patient and his parents back to a trauma room and just like that, the people in the waiting room closed in and swarmed the desk again.

I sat down and started registering patients while my coworker stood behind me.

"Is she gonna be okay?" asked one of our frequent flyers about the young lady.

I rolled my eyes. "She'll get through it."

And, you know, I sincerely believed that.

But then the girl started sobbing, and when I glanced at the security room mirror to shoot her another 'what is wrong with you?' look, I shit you not, she fainted and hit her head on our counter when she went down.

So, not only were we busy as hell with all of these people waiting to be seen, but my coworker was on the floor, bleeding; there was no triage nurse up front, and there were officially no beds open in the ER.

Cue the nervous laughter mixed with hints of irritation and a slight urge to throw my hands up in the air and walk out right then and there.

I called to the back to get help for my coworker and tried my best to calm the crowd in the lobby by registering them at lightning speed and pointing them toward the overflowing waiting room. I then started calling my coworkers to see if anyone could come in at a bit after 11 at night.

It wasn't a big surprise that most of my coworkers didn't answer the calls or they were busy with their families.

When I called my boss, I was met with the latter response, but he had the gall to ask of me, "Can you take [coworker's name] paperwork and a laptop to her bed and see if she can do anything while they take a look at her?"

Let your mouth hang open a minute.

I sighed and hung up.

As I was realizing how far up shit creek I was without a paddle, mom of the beat-up little boy came running out of the waiting room, screaming into her cell phone.

"That's your response?" she yelled. "You're telling me 'boys will be boys' is the reason your kid came in my yard and beat my son so badly he might be blind the rest of his life? You don't deserve to have kids."

I overheard a woman on the line yelling back, but the patient's mom furiously stabbed at the end call button before shoving her phone in her pocket. She started crying and was yanking tissues out of the box on the counter to the point that it would have made more sense for her to just take the whole box.

"Do you want me to call in someone for you to talk to?" I asked. "We have a pastor on call tonight, or sometimes a counselor can come down and help you through times like this."

She shook her head.

"That kid is two fucking years older than my son. My son calls him a friend, but we've had so much trouble with him that I was this close," she said, pinching her fingers together, "to telling the kid to stay out of my yard and away from my son. And then this happens."

I didn't have to really ask what happened because mom told me.

"I was in the shower while John was riding his bike in front of the house, and when I got out of the shower he was fine. I saw that kid was out there and yelled out the window for them to stay close to the house and not run off."

Mom explained the two had wandered off before to dangerous bodies of water in the area or entered abandoned, condemned houses. The mother said at one point, she found her son and the other kid sword fighting with sticks whittled to have razor-sharp tips. Her son had also recently been accused of stealing from a convenience store, but a quick look at the store's footage showed the other kid dropping candy in the pockets of the unsuspecting patient's backpack.

She then stated she was blow drying her hair when she heard a screech from her front yard, so she rushed to the window to see the older kid kicking her child in the face before grabbing a twig from the ground and hitting the boy in the eye with it.

Once the patient came to, he told a doctor, mental health duty officer, and Child Protective Services counselor the same story: the older kid wanted to take the patient's new bicycle, but the patient refused. After several minutes of trying to convince and then threaten the patient to give up his bike, the older kid grew frustrated and started beating the patient.

Based on the way the assailant's mother responded to the patient's mother's phone call, police were notified and the case was treated as a criminal act. The child had to be transferred out because he suffered an orbital fracture and doctors were unsure if the boy would be able to see out of his injured eye in the future. The patient also lost several of his adult teeth and sustained a jaw fracture during the assault, making an oral surgeon necessary. We learned the pre-teen had three broken fingers, a dislocated shoulder, and the lacerations to his cheeks and knees required 12 stiches.

My coworker was discharged around the time the little boy was flying out from our hospital, and she went home for the night.

I guess it would be fair to say she went home forever because she called the next day to tell us she wasn't cut out for this line of work and she was going to go back to working as a bookkeeper for her grandmother's business.

Hide and Seek

A very kind alcoholic well-known to hospital staff as well as the police department scuttled inside one night and didn't slow down to say a word to me.

Instead, he rushed in the waiting room and I watched on the security monitors how the guy knelt down and wiggled in between two chairs.

Hmmm.

I didn't wonder for too much longer because two cops showed up, took one look in the waiting room, and walked right up to the patient.

"We found you, John," one of the officers stated. "You can come on out from your little hiding spot."

Probably knowing he was on his way to jail again, our friendly frequent flyer slurred to the cops, "No, thank you. I'm quite comfortable where I am."

He was registered as a jail clearance and his BAC was over .5.

It's a Jungle Out There

I have a scar on my palm from childhood, that I sustained when I stupidly tried to remove a bone from a dog's mouth and the dog inadvertently went to chomp down on the bone but grabbed my hand instead. The wound was small, but deep. I think the moment I became interested in trauma was when I wiggled my thumb and could see the little white thing jumping around inside my hand.

In hindsight, I probably could or should have gone to the hospital for stitches, but I grew up in the era of 'suck it up, it's not that bad,' and 'yeah, that iodine/peroxide hurts, don't it?' My siblings and I didn't ride in booster seats; we fought over which of us got to sit in the front passenger seat, we rode our bikes down gravel hills while we weren't wearing helmets. We hiked through the woods with only each other and a big old dog that lived out back. We ate berries we picked along the dark path as we were coming in from the night.

But it's a different day and age now. Kids don't really go outside anymore—the ones here, at least. And when I do see kids outside, they're the ones I think need their parents the most because they're throwing rocks through home windows or screaming at passing cars or are out riding bikes down the middle of the road at three in the morning.

When I go out to shop, to the park, or even to work, I realize maybe I'm getting old because I find myself thinking things like, 'That sure wouldn't fly in my day,' or even saying things aloud like, 'If I talked to my mom like that when I was that girl's age, I wouldn't be here to tell you about it.'

Though many out there may disagree about teaching children manners or disciplining children or at what age (if any) a child should have a cell phone or a laptop or be allowed to walk to the park by him/herself, I'm going to step out of my position as a simple registration clerk to say we should all be teaching children about the proper behavior around animals, as well as the proper treatment of animals.

Now that I've taken a short trip down memory lane, I'll give you some examples of injuries caused in animal-related incidents that our patients (mostly children) have registered with over the years.

- A teen was brought in by ambulance because the two Great Danes the family had owned for four years attacked the boy. As the night went on and he was receiving sutures to both forearms, we learned the boy had been abusing the dogs by inviting his friends over to feed the dogs drugs. While the dogs were high, the group of teens would take turns physically abusing the dogs and posting the pictures online. One night, I guess both dogs just snapped. Luckily, for the teen, his parents were home and dragged the dogs off of him. He was arrested for animal abuse, but I think the judge agreed the stitches up and down the

boy's arms were enough of a
punishment.

- Sometimes injuries happen just
  because parents do stupid things and
  care more about their own needs than
  protecting their kid, like in the case of
  the barely-walking toddler brought in
  by ambulance because porcupine
  needles were jammed in her face, upper
  chest wall, and upper arms. I guess her
  dad bought the animal at an exotic
  animal auction and owned the thing for
  less than a week before the incident.
  Around this time, I think a bear
  attacked someone upstate, and then
  Ohio started rethinking its rules for
  exotic pets.

- Another young child was attacked by a
  rabid raccoon because his caretakers
  didn't recognize the signs of rabies.
  When the animal approached their
  riverside campsite, they encouraged the
  boy to meet the animal for a picture
  opportunity, and the boy had to get

stitches to his shoulder and calf. In addition to this, the child had to receive a round of shots to deal with the rabies. We knew it tested positive because the boy's uncle had a gun in the tent and killed the raccoon once it attacked. He brought the animal to us in one of those little red coolers.

- An adult man said the 118-pound dog he adopted from the shelter 'had an attitude problem' and kept 'mean-mugging' him, so the man sat cross legged on the floor in front of the dog and stared the animal in the eyes. If you have an experience with dogs…or a lot of animals, really…you'll know this can prove to be highly dangerous, as some animals will view this as an act of aggression. In this case, the man's new dog did just that, and the animal responded by lunging forward and biting the man in the face. It wasn't just a simple chomp down and go bite, however. The tip of the man's nose was gone. GONE. He was covered in blood and we could see every muscle, tendon…whatever those things were that make up the human nose. We knew he had to be flown out before he even arrived at the hospital based on the report from the medics. The dog was NOT harmed in this case. Although the man told medics 'just kill it,' one of the medics took it upon herself to adopt the dog. The elderly animal lived out the rest of its life peacefully and never had another biting incident. By the way, the patient's BAC was about .35.

- Around holidays, I think you'll notice ads in newspapers or on TV that warn against adopting animals based on holidays, like ones urging parents not to buy their kids rabbits for Easter. I wish people also knew not to buy animals based on the animals in movies. A few years ago, someone bought a Neapolitan Mastiff because they saw the breed in the *Harry Potter* movies. Dog owners know that dogs need training and generally know you can't buy a dog, let it run loose, and then expect the animal to know the difference between right and wrong. In this case, the owner did not train the not-so-gentle giant, nor did he socialize the animal. On several occasions, the animal got out and killed neighbors' cats, chickens, and generally did what dogs do: spent its time out looking for prey and play. After a warning from the cops to secure the dog's surroundings, the owner failed to comply. The dog escaped once more and bit a child who was skateboarding down the road. We think the dog was trying to play with the child more than he was trying to hurt her because she only had one bite to her skin, and it was a shallow bite that we found under her ripped sweatshirt and under-shirt. However, during the time the girl was trying to get away from the dog, she fell against the road and busted her nose open and broke one of her teeth. It wasn't a great night to be in the ER, with that child screaming bloody murder while doctors stitched her up. The patient's family didn't blame the dog for this, and as a pet owner, I'm glad about that. The dog's owner was ticketed and the dog was taken by authorities to be destroyed. There's good news, though! The dog was instead placed with an out-of-state rescue organization for the breed and we hear it had to go through obedience training before being placed in a home with no small animals, other dogs, or small children.

- I've been employed with the hospital for several years and can say I have only seen three injuries caused by Pit Bulls. Two were viewed on our reports of daily chief complaints, and one was viewed in person. The patient I registered was playing with his dogs in the yard and tried to be sneaky and hide their squeaky toy down his pants. One of the dogs knocked him over and the other bit his ass cheek. The man was crying because he was embarrassed, and he said no to our hospital directory because he didn't want anyone to know he was at the hospital. He didn't punish the pets; he knew what he did was dumb.

- Box turtles and snapping turtles are far from the same thing, and it's a shame the parent to the pre-teen couldn't explain that to the boy beforehand. I don't have any idea what doctors did to get the small spiked turtle to release its grip on the boy's hand, but I do know the kid lost two fingers to this accident. He blamed his mom because she allegedly told him, 'Go on, you can pick it up.'

- If you live in the country, you're probably aware of what a pig scramble is, and if not, it's fairly simple. See, a certain number of children are chosen to chase a number of piglets through an enclosed pen. There are fewer piglets than children, and the object of this event is to be one of the children to catch a pig. It's pretty entertaining because pigs are pretty quick and the second you lift them they sound like baby Mandrakes. (Yep, going with Potter references during this book.) One piglet apparently didn't take kindly to being chased and yanked by the legs, so it whipped its head around and somehow bit a little boy on the abdomen. The tiny cowboy was brought in and patched up. Throughout his ER visit, he didn't cry once. He was too busy flirting with all of the nurses and telling them about how he caught a piglet and how excited he was to take it home.

- I'm sure we can all agree that cats are furry assholes, running around the house at all hours, plotting their owners' deaths. In this case, we started to believe this was nothing but the truth because a woman came in to get stitches to her forehead, cheeks, nose, and lips. While she was sleeping, her cat jumped from the bed to the ceiling fan, which then fell from the ceiling and hit the sleeping woman in the face. The globes and the light bulbs shattered against her skin. I think she ended up with something like 30 stitches and then had to take the cat to the vet for a checkup.

A crying, hysterical father brought his exceptionally calm—but extremely bloody—toddler to the desk.

"What happened?" I asked.

"He cut his dingy off! He found a pair of scissors and just cut it off! My wife walked in and found him playing in the blood."

If I was reading this book, I was surely question this story, but the boy's penis was severed. His wife brought the child's appendage inside, kept in a Ziploc bag filled with ice.

The little boy was transferred to a pediatric hospital and the only time I heard him cry is when lab went in the room.

That's one of the strangest things I've ever encountered in the ER.

A Message to Readers:

Thanks for taking time out of your hectic life to check out this book. I hope you've found it entertaining and worth your time.

Now, this is the first time I've tried a NSFW edition, and I'm not sure I'll do it again. While it's been great to blow off steam and tell stories a little differently than I tell them in my 'clean' editions, I think all the dirty words are best saved for telling the stories in person because I'm not so sure the humor I'm trying to pass on through this language shines through as much as it makes me seem like an insensitive jerk. For this reason, and to offer the same clean entertainment to readers who'd rather not deal with that language or dark humor, I've made the choice to offer this NSFW edition as a clean version, though some of the one-page stories may only be included within the edition you're viewing because they're simply too dirty and short to break down for the clean book.

As I've said before, I type up all of my books—and I usually do this after extremely long shifts, right before I go to bed. Even when I'm off work and editing, I miss stuff. I read things how I think they should be, not what they are. I am extremely grateful to readers for leaving me reviews with typos. In order to fix these typos, I have pull my books from Amazon, and then they're not available to readers. I want to offer the best product to readers, but at the same time, some of my books won't be available while I'm fixing errors. So, basically, I have to choose carefully when I want to do this. I do, however, have a list of typos to go back through and edit to offer you the best quality for the price you paid.

I cannot express how grateful I am to loyal readers. Some of you have left reviews for each edition of the series, and I see them. I'm shouting out a big THANK YOU!!!!!!! to you because without you I'd probably go crazy without something to do with all these stories trapped in my head. Seriously, I can't thank you enough. I love all of my readers and only wish to offer you the best account I can of

109

what I've seen, and I can't thank you all enough for reading.

As to answer a few questions/respond to reviews, I'll go ahead and do that now.

One, I can't tell you exactly how I gained permission to write these books or if I did. I can't give details about any of that process. However, I can tell you none of the details about these patients match exact details. I try to write these stories while saving the patient's personality, but I value patient privacy and will never cross the boundaries of privacy by exposing patient identifiers to readers. In addition, I have altered some of the dialogue and details of the stories if I feel they are too easy for non-medical staff to identify. Several of these stories can be found in news sources online, but I try to avoid using too much information so that you could do that because that's still breeching patient privacy.

Someone kind of blasted me for a few phrases I use in the book. I guess the reader has or had experience in the medical field. I'm not a nurse or a doctor or any certified medical professional, and I'll be the first one to say that. There are so many things about the medical field that I don't know. I just call them what I see or am told they are. What I know about a stemi is that it's a procedure when the patient goes to the Cath Lab and the arteries are cleared or a stent is placed by accessing the area through the patient's groin…from what people have explained to me. Maybe that's wrong, I don't know. Maybe I explained it wrong, I don't know. I also didn't have any idea like 'everyone knows' that patients don't 'flat line' in the ER. I've been standing in rooms or right outside of them or in the nurses' station when monitors have stopped steadily beeping and have gone flat. If I'm not using the right term, sorry. So, in a way, I DO apologize for any misinformation I offer to readers, but at the same time, I'm kind of doing the best I can to explain what I've seen just based on what I've seen with no medical training. No harm, no foul…I mean, that's what I'd hope, but that's not always the case.

If you have any questions or concerns, please don't hesitate to leave a review. I'll do the best I can to answer questions, and typos are definitely noted!

Have a great day!

Check me out on Twitter!

https://twitter.com/AuthorKerryHamm

Made in the USA
Columbia, SC
10 December 2017